Cardiovascular Health and You

What You Need to Know Before It Is Too Late!

RON KNESS

Published By

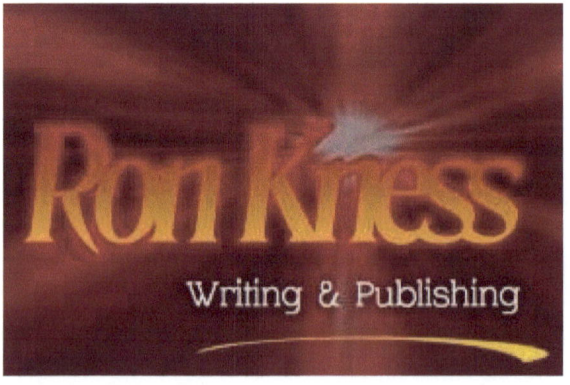

Copyright © 2017 Ron Kness

All rights reserved.

ISBN-13: 978-1548004620
ISBN-10: 1548004626

Contents

Disclaimer

This publication is for informational purposes only and is not intended as medical advice. Medical advice should always be obtained from a qualified medical professional for any health conditions or symptoms associated with them.

Every possible effort has been made in preparing and researching this material. We make no warranties with respect to the accuracy, applicability of its contents or any omissions.

See your healthcare professional before starting any diet, health or exercise program!

Introduction

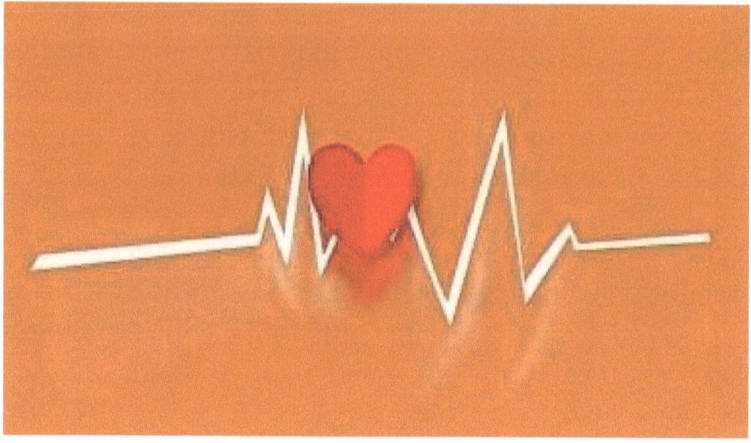

In the United States, one of the leading causes of death is heart disease. Heart disease should not be taken lightly though, since it is considered the top killer for both men and women in many countries around the word, especially in America. According to its definition, heart disease is a medical condition in which the heart and the blood vessels are affected. This term also refers to a number of diseases that affect the heart including:

> ➢ arterial fibrillation

> ➢ heart attack

> ➢ coronary artery disease

> ➢ heart valve disease

Getting diagnosed for it is indeed quite alarming, but catching it early can minimize or even reverse the effects of the disease.

Better yet is preventing it in the first place through a healthy lifestyle.

Heart disease is prevalent in lots of developed countries and many experts attribute it to certain environmental factors. The good news about this type of disease is that, it can be prevented by following certain healthy living practices.

Although heart disease is indeed one of the top causes for untimely deaths in America, a person diagnosed with it should not consider it as a death sentence. There are actually lots of cases when a heart disease can still be treated or reversed, as long as proper steps are taken, and the person involved is disciplined and persistent enough in achieving their goals.

Preventing heart disease can be done in a lot of ways, all which will point out to living a healthier life. Thus, it basically means that you may have to make some changes in your own lifestyle today, in order to achieve it. If some of your relatives have been diagnosed for certain types of heart disease, then it is best that you visit your doctor regularly. Regular checkups would really help a lot aside from the fact that doctors are the best persons to know what needs to be done in order to prevent it.

By visiting your doctor, s/he would be able to tell your risk level as far as getting affected by heart disease is concerned, through your blood pressure, cholesterol, fibrinogen, triglycerides and homocysteine levels.

Aside from visiting your doctor on a regular basis, there are also certain things that you can do on your own to prevent it; one of which is following a proper diet.

A healthy diet is something that should be low in saturated fat, refined sugar, and cholesterol. Aside from that, you should also make sure that you provide your body with adequate amounts of vitamins, minerals, and dietary fiber.

Healthy living means that you should quit smoking and alcohol drinking soon. Getting enough exercise should also be included in your health plan, and it is also important to provide your body with enough rest. By taking note of these important facts about heart disease, you should be able to come up with your own plan, which will help you in preventing it from affecting your life.

Different Types of Cardiovascular Disease

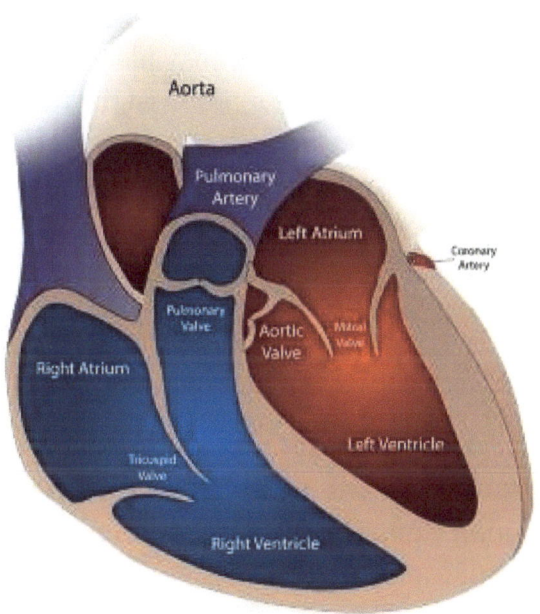

As noted, cardiovascular disease has become among the leading causes of death around the world. With unhealthy eating and lifestyle choices becoming more common, education about what kinds of diseases will become more important. Alternatively, there are a number of conditions that are genetic or inborn conditions. What are the primary cardiovascular diseases out there?

This chapter will be covering this topic along with some broad descriptions and causes and things you can do in your life to minimize the risk of getting heart disease.

Coronary Artery Disease (CAD)

The appearance of coronary artery disease is usually characterized by the hardening or shrinking of the pathways in coronary arteries. This creates easy places for blockages to form and restrict the passage of blood to the heart. This condition is the most common cause of heart attack, and strokes. Leaving this process unchecked will undoubtedly end in death.

Heart Attack

Heart attack is a broad term for conditions that restrict or completely cut off blood flow; medically, it is termed myocardial infarction. The most common cause for heart attack is the buildup of arterial plaque formed by free-floating cholesterol in the blood that collects in areas where it can solidify into a mass which eventually blocks the passageways of the blood and stops the flow. Some people are born with defects that can cause them to have sudden heart attacks when older such as arteries that develop twisted.

Arrhythmia

This is simply a term for any sudden change to the normal rhythm of the heartbeat. The issue with this condition is that it is of an electrical nature rather than a physical one. What happens, is that electrical impulses that control the heartbeat begin to become confused, or out of order. When this takes place, the heart beats in an irregular fashion which can cause damage to other organs that require a steady flow of blood to function properly.

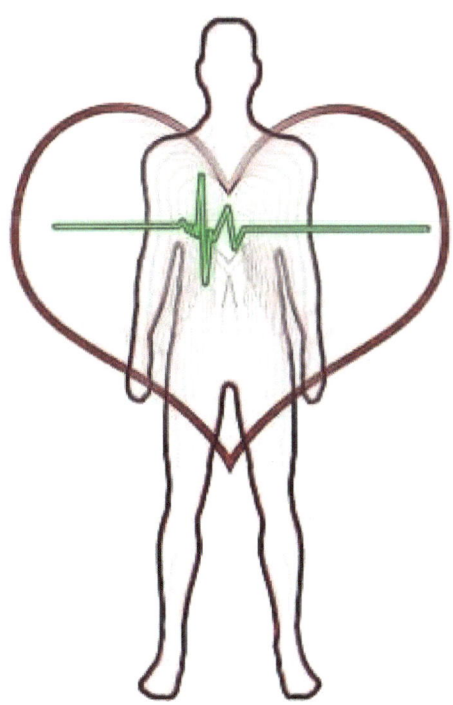

Heart Failure

Isn't the same as a heart attack in that instead of the heart stopping suddenly, the heart simply doesn't pump enough blood for the body to function properly. When organs aren't fed enough blood and oxygen, they can shut down resulting in a feeling of loss of breath. Some people can live with this for a period of time before realizing the seriousness of the symptoms, which usually manifest in the general form of fatigue.

If you have risk factors for any of these cardiovascular diseases, it is important to seek out treatment right away.

Are You at Risk For Cardiovascular Disease?

If you're not aware of the factors that could increase your risk for heart disease, heart issues could suddenly appear without warning. It's important to realize that by increasing your awareness, and knowing what you can do to protect yourself by recognizing the signs associated with heart problems, could save your life or the lives of other around you. Since this topic is relatively nuanced, it'll be good to look at each of the factors as they affect people across demographics. The following will contain a few of the factors that put you at risk for cardiovascular disease.

Things You Can't Change

There are a number of factors that are encoded in genetics that there is little you can do about. If your family has a history of heart problems or defects, then it is possible for you to experience some issues with at that as you get older. Age is another factor that is relatively inevitable, because as your age increases, so do your chances of heart issues. Men are generally at the highest risk when age and family history are in the mix, but women who are post-menopausal are also considered to be a part of the high risk group.

What You Can Change

Even though there are many things beyond your control, there are still quite a few things that you can do to safeguard yourself against heart issues. This can be done by choosing to avoid specific habits, and engaging in healthy practices (and not in unhealthy ones).

Smoking is considered one of the most dangerous in this group because of its vein and artery-restricting effect on your vascular system. This condition can lead to the easy formation of blood clots and increase blood pressure to dangerous levels. When your heart has to work harder to push the blood through restricted vessels, it can easily become tired and fail.

Being Overweight

When you are overweight, this is another factor that can put a hefty strain on your cardiovascular system. Large amount of body fat makes it more difficult for your heart to beat without massive amounts of stress. It also makes it far more difficult to breathe. When breathing becomes more shallow, it can put your body into fight or flight mode, putting even more strain on an already struggling heart. The best thing to do is avoid any of the bad choices that will contribute to an already burdened cardiovascular system, such as stopping smoking and losing weight ... but there is even more you can do!

Easy Ways to Reduce Stress

Another factor that increases the risk of heart disease is excessive stress. Through past research, we know that the effects of excessive stress can manifest itself in a number of physical ways in addition to the known mental ones.

Here are three ways you can reduce stress that will lighten the load on your heart.

Deep Breathing Exercise Is Valuable

When was the last time you thought seriously and focused all of your efforts on your breathing? Studies have shown that deep breathing exercises have a calming effect on the body and can help to fight anxiety that can choke out your inner peace. Slow controlled breaths will reduce your heart rate and get you out of fight or flight mode. Taking the time to sit off to the side of situations and focus on your breathing can bring a lot of focus and help you to solve problems that might make you feel as if your world is ending.

A Little Bit of Workout

When stress is building in your mind, it can manifest itself in a multitude of muscle pain and stiffness because of the release of certain hormones and a natural tendency to clench. Because of this, pent up energy caused by stress places a strain on your body, both mentally and physically.

A great way to relieve this pent up energy is to release it through exercise. Finding a healthy way to channel excess energies can help you to cope with stress on both a psychological and a physical level by showing that you really can achieve control by relieving pent up energy through working out.

Eat Healthy Food

The human body needs to eat to live, much the way that any machine runs on some kind of fuel. In order to have a healthy happy body, it's paramount to feed your body the kind of food that fosters efficient, fully-functional day-to-day health. Balanced nutrition means your mind is more likely to produce the chemicals known to regulate stress hormones and mood. That way, when you reach the end of your day, your body will be ready for another night of regenerative sleep.

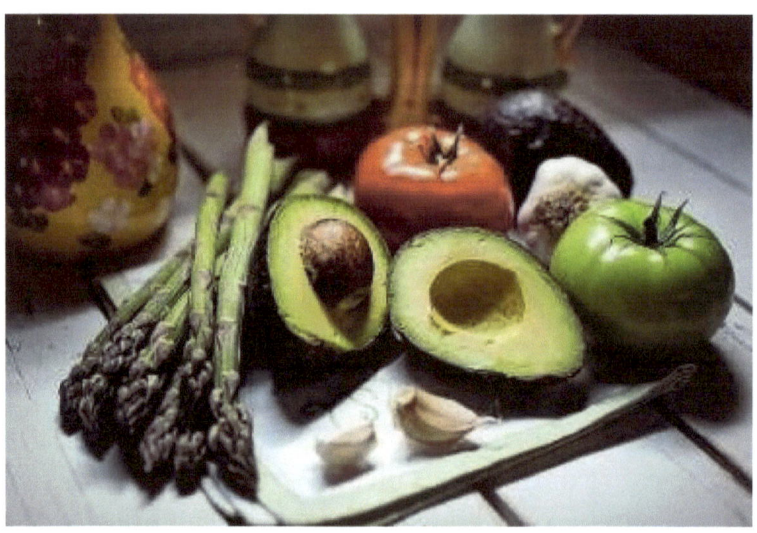

Deep breathing, exercising and eating a healthy diet are three easy ways to reduce stress and it insidious effects. Try them all and see if you don't feel better in the end.

Common Risk Factors For a Stroke

Strokes can cause a number of debilitating effects that can last for lifetime. Even with modern medicine being on the cutting edge of discovering cures and treatments, the need to focus on preventative care still needs to be addressed. When you look at the collection of factors that surround a health issue, it is always easier to safeguard yourself, or at least reduce the appearance of negative health events. Here is a short list of common risk factors for a stroke.

Family History

When a family member before you has heart disease, not related to external causes, such as unhealthy eating, obesity or smoking, it increases your chances of having some kind of heart-related health event too. This is because a person related to you will have similar genetics, and therefore you will carry many of the same developmental DNA genetics in your system, including defects that can increase your chances of having a heart-related event. This makes it easier for doctors to know what to look for when you go get an annual checkup. That can rule out diseases and make it easier to find the cause of symptoms that are more particular to you, or pinpoint the exact source of the problem before it becomes a life-threatening issue.

Atrial Fibrillation

If your heart is prone to arrhythmic activity, you are at a much higher risk of stroke, because poor blood flow can cause blood clots and other blood obstructions. Sometimes during one of these episodes, a person will experience pain in their chest that can be very startling. If the heart is weak, then it may not be able to get enough blood to other important organs like the brain, which can result in dizzy spells and tiredness. When this kind of disruption continues for a sustained amount of time it can result in serious damage to the heart and make it harder for you to breathe.

Transient Ischemic Attack

This condition can manifest itself in a few different ways, and they are generally considered to be more serious signs of what could be the first signs of an increased likelihood of a stroke. When you feel faint, dizzy or confused to the degree that you are having trouble thinking. If you have a hard time swallowing or your ability to feel sensation in your fingertips has lessened. Weakness on one side of the body is another clue, and the one of the most frightening of these is loss of the ability to engage in coherent speech.

The Tell-Tale Signs

One of the most telling signs that you are going to probably have a stroke are transient ischemic attacks. This happens when a small blood clot blocks a passageway to the brain and the brain begins to malfunction due to a lack of blood. Below are a few examples of TIA that can accurately foreshadow the possibility that you are likely to have a stroke as soon as in a few hours:

- **Slurred Speech** - The most immediately recognizable sign that you are going to have a stroke is when you begin to have difficulty speaking. Cases of slurred speech have been well documented, often happening in the middle of a sentence. This can be very jarring to people near the sufferer and if a person is unaware that slurred speech or incoherent babbling are a sign of a stroke, then precious time may be lost until the person receives medical attention. Studies have shown that those receiving medical attention at a hospital within one hour of showing symptoms have a better rate of recovery.

- **Sudden Confusion** - Aside from slurred speech, it is possible to become confused to the point of not being able to recall information that is well known to you, such as your place of residence or your job. This temporary condition is a serious sign of impending stroke, and should be handled with patience and care. When someone is disoriented, it won't accomplish anything to badger them for details. The first priority is always to get them medical attention as soon as possible.

- **Weakness on One Side** - This takes place when a blood clot is lodged in some part of the circulatory system and blocking the blood flow to the brain especially to the part of the brain that controls that side from operating at full efficiency – thus the weakness. This causes the signals sent from the brain to be weaker than normal, and in much the same way, weakens the response to the command sent.

The Dangers of High Cholesterol

Even though the particles of cholesterol in the blood are very small, they have the ability to pose a massive problem to any person who is dealing with other health issues. High cholesterol has become a common thing among adult men, so it is worth discussing the fact that it can lead to life threatening conditions that negatively affect your cardiovascular system, but what are these dangers? Continue reading to find out the breakdown of the dangers of high cholesterol.

High Blood Pressure

Issues with cholesterol can begin in a relatively reversible, benign way, but over time problems can develop. One of these problems, is that blood with a high concentration of cholesterol can eventually experience a settling of the cholesterol, where the particles stick to the walls of veins and arteries.

As the particles collect, they will begin to obstruct the vital pathways of blood, and prevent blood from reaching sensitive areas with a variety of outcomes – most of which are not good. This can be especially deadly if you are a person that happens to have a birth defect in some part of your coronary artery, or another essential place in your circulatory system that can make it an easy target for plaque accumulation.

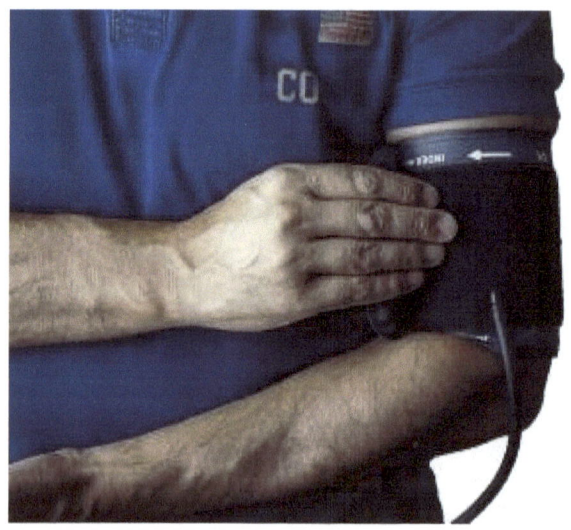

Stroke

As noted before, strokes are the result of a blockage in some part of the circulatory system that leads to the brain. This can lead to a variety of different issues, but in some cases, it's possible for blood to be cut off from the parts of the brain that control essential functions of the body like the heart, or lungs. Most of the time however, it results in some form of paralysis or loss of motor function in some part of the body.

Some common stroke involve loss of feeling in the arm, or the loss of muscular control in the left side of the face.

Heart Attack

This is definitely the most serious of these conditions. A heart attack is usually any time that the blood flow is cut off from, or restricted to the heart to the point of being life threatening. When this takes place, it can cause scarring damage to the arteries and veins around the heart. This usually means that the chances of another heart attack are higher, and could easily result in death. This is particularly dangerous when it occurs due to blockage in the coronary artery.

Signs You Might Be Having a Heart Attack

Even though heart attacks are fairly common, and a lot of people these days survive them, there is still a wide gap between actual knowledge about heart attacks, and what the public largely gleaned from movies. Real heart attacks are often more difficult to detect, and can appear in very subtle ways. Knowing these signs could save your life, so this chapter explores just a few of the signs that you might be having a heart attack.

Common Symptoms

When someone is beginning to have a heart attack, it's not always clear that a heart attack is what is happening. Some people may have a range of symptoms and not others. Some these include the chest tightness, or heavy feeling and discomfort. Sometimes this discomfort can go away and then return suddenly. You might experience pain that radiates from the chest and out into extremities or limbs. This is often accompanied by a shortness of breath, or breaking out in a cold sweat. You could experience nausea or lightheadedness. This often happens because blood is having difficulty reaching its destination in the body.

In Women

It's important to take note that women can experience heart attack without any chest tightness. It's common for them to dismiss discomfort or limb numbness as related to something else. Because symptoms in women can be different than men, and not as commonly discussed, pay very close attention to your body and know the signs of heart attack in women.

The Cough

In itself, a cough usually doesn't mean anything serious, but there a few things that it would be a very good idea to watch. This is especially true if you are a person who has been diagnosed with some form of heart disease, or if you are in the high-risk category. If you have a cough that won't quit, and you have white or pinkish mucus coming up, then that could very well be a sign of heart failure. When the heart is too weak to pump blood properly, blood leaks into your lungs, then irritating the lungs and coloring the mucus. If you have these symptoms, it's important to contact your doctor immediately.

Act Quickly For The Best Outcome

No matter who is suffering these symptoms, it's important to act quickly before things escalate. As soon as symptoms appear, call your emergency service. If the person in question loses consciousness, every minute counts.

Important Steps That Reduce Your Risk For Heart Attack

Heart-related issues have risen in the last few decades in the cause of death among men. While there are many different details and issues surrounding these situations, it's clear that a portion of it could have been avoided due to certain lifestyle changes that promote a healthier potential for living as you grow older. What kinds of things can you do to help yourself avoid possible illness? Here are some important steps that reduce your risk for heart attack.

Get Active Today

One of the most important parts of being healthy is having some kind of activity in your week. Many studies that have done research on exercise have shown that any person doing exercise three or more times a week greatly reduces the risk of heart-related issues and problems. Physical activity helps lower high blood pressure and clear free-floating fats from your bloodstream that could build up and cause blood clots leading to stroke or heart failure. It has been noted that any sort of exercise is better than none at all, and anything that gets the heart rate up can help to strengthen the heart, and thus provide a small extended health benefit for the person exercising.

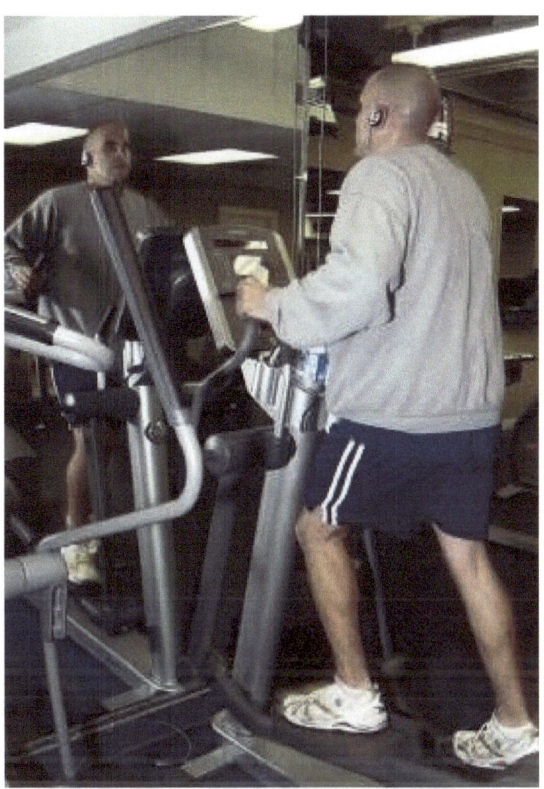

Healthy Nutrition

One the other most important things that you can do for your body is to be sure that you are getting the healthiest, freshest and most balanced nutrition possible. Foods that contain the nutrients that your body needs will fill your body with the building blocks of what it needs to make repairs, build and replace new cells and carry out a multitude of other important bodily functions. If you make a regular practice of ingesting things that aren't healthy for your body, you will be rebuilt with these bad ingredients. Be sure to choose foods that are healthy; natural or organic is even better. In other words, you literally are what you eat!

Keep Your Weight Under Control

Being overweight is one of the most consistent predictors of heart issues. When you gain weight, a lot of problems can occur, especially issues with the passageways leading to the heart. If the cholesterol in your blood settles in the nooks of your arteries, that could spell trouble very quickly, because an obstructed artery can lead to stroke or heart attack, so it's important to eat right, and keep up with exercise to avoid gaining weight. When fat builds up around your heart, it makes it work harder, thus increasing the risk of heart failure.

You may have noticed these three recommendations of exercising, eating healthy and losing weight are not new. Yet, Americans continue to be the fattest nation in the world, so people are not heeding the advice. Why make your loved ones suffer needlessly because you did not heed these simple three thongs that could have prevented your heart-related event that left you either disabled or dead.

Hypertension 101

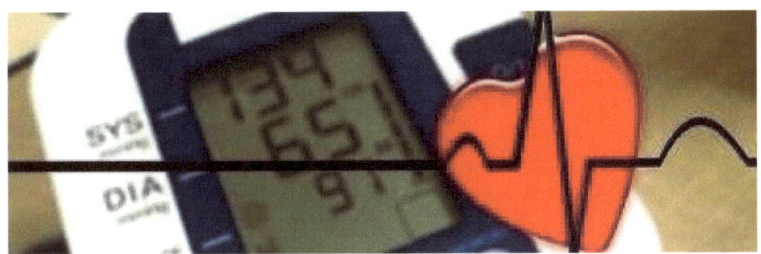

After the last chapter, you are aware of needing to eat right, exercise, and maintain a proper weight, but this isn't just recommended for general health and wellness. It is also essential because it helps you to improve your cardiovascular health. Most people only get one heart in their life, so why would you not want to take care of it!

What is cardiovascular health? This is the health status of your heart, arteries, veins and other parts that make up your cardiovascular system which all work together to provide you with life. When your cardio health starts to decline, it puts you at risk for heart disease and stroke, both of which can be fatal.

A big part of your maintaining good cardiovascular health is looking for signs that it could be declining, such as with hypertension. Hypertension is something not to be messed around with. Here are some things to know about hypertension and what can be done about it.

1. What is Hypertension?

When discussing hypertension, it's important to recognize specific facts that can clearly define what it is, how it is measured, and how it can affect your health. In recent years, it has become a more common condition, so the need for information on it has become far greater than previously required.

Before you can find out if you could be at risk, or suffering from this condition, it is necessary to know the numbers, so the following is an explanation of what defines hypertension.

What Is It Exactly

Hypertension is a cardiovascular disease that is more widely known by its common name, high blood pressure. You are said to have hypertension when your heart has to work harder to pump blood through your arteries and veins.

This is often caused by some form of restriction of blood flow due to either the heavy presence of blood borne fat, or by the actual physical constriction of the blood vessels. Either way, this condition can lead to more serious, and possibly life-threatening issues if left unchecked.

Measuring Hypertension

When you are getting your blood pressure checked, the most common healthy levels should be under 120 systolic and under 80 diastolic. Commonly known as 120/80 or 120 over 80. If you haven't been monitoring your blood pressure, and it's beginning to become unhealthy, you may find your numbers in a higher range, such as 140-159 systolic or 90-99 diastolic.

This is considered to be stage 1 high blood pressure. If you are at 160 and above systolic or 100 or above diastolic, you would be considered stage 2 blood pressure. Anything above 180 systolic or above 110 diastolic would be considered a life-threatening emergency, or hypertensive crisis.

2. What Are the Potential Causes?

Despite what was previously believed, a person can live with hypertension for quite some time without exhibiting any form of symptoms; it really depends on your numbers. In order to safeguard yourself or loved ones from the effects of hypertension, it is important to learn the potential causes of hypertension.

It's a good idea to take note of any similarities in your experience as you read the rest of this chapter.

A Glitch In Your Genetics

Over the last few decades, science has begun to finally be able to detangle the threads of DNA to discover what kinds of illnesses or conditions each person may be predisposed to during their life. Before that, the doctor's best way to narrow down the list of possible causes for ailments came in the form of simply asking what health problems are common to their family members.

This knowledge allowed them to make better guesses about treatments and eliminate solutions that are unlikely to be of any help of the cause was genetic-related.

Your Habits

If you drink or smoke, you will be at higher risk for hypertension - period. And especially if you engage in both activities. Smoking contributes heavily to the hardening of the arteries, and hard arteries don't flex as much which exponentially raise the chances of life-threatening strokes.

This is because arteries that burst are much harder to fix than arteries that have blockage. A hemorrhaging artery in or near the brain is likely to kill you immediately.

Not Enough Activity

A sedentary lifestyle can be one of the worst things for high blood pressure. When you aren't active enough, the fluids in your blood that pump through your body to help cleanse it, such as lymph, are unable to carry toxins, wastes and other undesirable matter to disposal sites within your body.

Arteries lose their elasticity when you don't move enough, and it can also lead to the slow buildup of arterial plaque from unchecked cholesterol.

3. What Signs and Symptoms Are There?

If not controlled, hypertension is a sign of impending health problems for the people who experience it, but before it progresses into more serious issues, there are often a collection of negative effects that signal the coming problems.

If you or a family member began to experience some of these symptoms without knowing how they are tied to your health, it could be easy to pass over these warning signs and unknowingly elevate yourself into a higher category of risk for a future cardiac event. Keep reading to know the signs.

Sometimes There Are No Signs

In previous decades, doctors made the incorrect assumption that hypertension was something that was always symptomatic, but more recent discoveries have revealed that you may not be able to detect hypertension with actually getting checked out.

This is a time when it's a good idea to take a look at your family history to see if you have any family members that suffer from this condition. If you have a parent, uncle, or grandparent that has dealt with hypertension, the likelihood that you are susceptible is extremely high.

Your Hearing Changes Suddenly

Have you ever been sitting and relaxing quietly when your hearing suddenly drops out for a moment? A lot of times that can be a sign that your blood pressure has changed. When you heart has to work extra hard to force blood through your blood vessels, the extra pressure it exerts can place extra strain on your ear drum making it less sensitive for a moment.

Fatty plaque can also become trapped in the tiny blood vessels of your ears, making hearing loss a more permanent experience.

Headaches, Head Rush, or Blurry Vision

Sometimes when you get up too fast, you may get slightly light headed. This can be a normal occurrence for many people, but if it's happening often, then you should get your blood pressure checked. When you are stationary, blood pools wherever it can sit. This means that when you stand, the blood will rush to reposition itself in your body, then creating the somewhat unpleasant sensation.

This can cause headaches or blurry vision depending on the health of your arteries. If you have experienced any of these types of issues, it would be a good idea to get checked out.

4. Are There Treatment Options?

Most people will be happy to know that there are a range of treatment options for those suffering from high blood pressure. While there are medicines available through a prescription from your doctor, there are also several natural foods that can help.

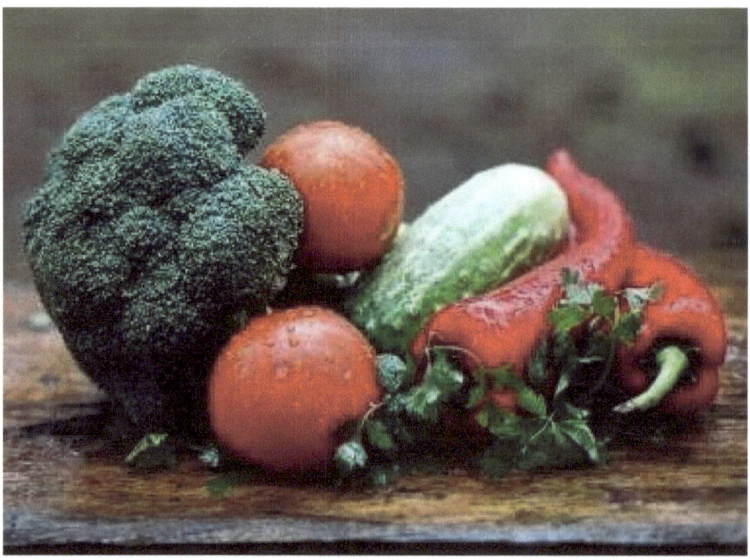

The best part about many of these natural treatments though, is that there are little to no side effects, so you have fewer chances of a bad reaction.

Fish Oil

This oil is very high in omega 3 fatty acids. These amazing antioxidant rich capsules help your veins and arteries to stay elastic, and the fatty acids help to break down deposits of plaque and cholesterol. One or two a day can significantly impact your cholesterol and help the body to eliminate free floating saturated fats.

Green Tea

Tea is an antioxidant rich drink that can help you to improve your health over time. Studies have shown that people who consumed two cups of tea a day were able to significantly improve their cholesterol levels. Green tea is also anti-inflammatory, and can help relax and widen irritated arteries. One study was able to see that after three weeks of tea consumption, arterial diameter was nearly doubled.

Lycopene

Although you can find lycopene in nearly any fruit or vegetable, tomatoes are currently known to have the highest concentration of this amazing chemical. Lycopene research has concluded that lycopene was extremely effective at breaking down dangerous blockages and deposits of fat in the arteries. This makes it an excellent way to prevent stroke and reduce the chance of a heart attack.

Garlic

For at least 2,000 years, garlic has been used in medicines and remedies of all different kinds. Today we realize that it's properties and benefits go far beyond flavoring our food. Garlic is now well known for its ability to lower triglycerides and cholesterol in the blood.

5. Can Hypertension Be Treated Naturally?

With the alarming number of people looking for alternatives to current approaches to medical conditions, more information about natural methods for treatment of illnesses has become widely available.

Much to the surprise of some, many of the treatments have turned out to be very useful in fighting the illnesses that they've been created for, and some of them have turned out to not only be rooted in history, but also science. The purpose of this paragraph is to share a few ways that hypertension can be treated naturally.

Get Some Exercise

When you exercise, several things happen. First of all, the movement from the exercise helps increase your circulation. This means that the blood flow to your body is increasing, making it easier to feed your organs and extremities.

Secondly, your heart rate increases, so your heart is beginning to get a workout by actively pushing it to its safe limits. This will help your heart to perform on a higher and more efficient level when you are at rest.

Lastly, this also helps your body to carry toxins and other impurities to disposal sites in your circulatory system.

Further, studies have shown that a person who engages in more physical activity lowers the potential for cardiac incidents.

Be Sure to Get Good Nutrition

Eating a healthier diet that consists of unsaturated fats and avoids trans fats, saturated fats, and processed forms of sugars will help you to stay healthy. These heavy saturated fats can raise your cholesterol to the point that makes it easy for you to get blood clots and arterial blockages that contribute to various forms of heart disease.

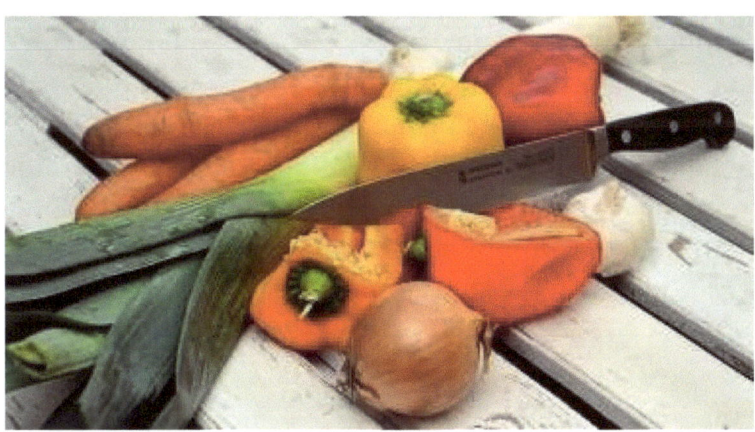

More On Saturated Fats

As noted, a great way to help avoid high blood pressure is to replace saturated fats with healthier unsaturated plant fats.

The unsaturated type are easier for the body to absorb and have a wide range of health benefits related to the heart and blood pressure. Because of the benefits, cutting back in saturated fats and replacing them with the unsaturated type lessens the amount of work that your heart has to do and gives you less of a chance for any kind of buildup.

Once again we see exercise and nutrition as two of the leading natural treatments to lower hypertension.

Eating fruits that contain lycopene can also help you to break down any potential for these blockages which can lead to strokes or heart attack. Healthy diet and exercise complement each other perfectly to help safeguard you from incidents.

Stop Smoking

The inhalation of smoke can contribute massively to the shrinking of arterial walls. This means that your heart has to work much harder to force blood through your circulatory system, and this not only puts extra strain on the organ, but also makes it easier for clots and blockages to form. These can lead to anything from benign temporary issues to more serious cardiac emergencies. Quitting smoking will allow your arteries to regain their natural elasticity.

Foods That Are Good For the Heart

Humans have been eating variations of similar foods for thousands of years. In recent times, science has discovered how many of these nutrient specific foods have been an integral part of human development and health all along, and why they help us to stay alive so well. There are many organs that are benefitted by nature's gifts, but which ones have the ability to help the heart? As you continue reading you will find a short list of foods that you should be eating to have good heart health.

Nuts

Nuts are high in a kind of fat that is very beneficial to the body. These kinds of fats are called unsaturated fats and have shown to reduce the chance of heart disease. That doesn't mean eating more of them than recommended is good, because health is achieved primarily through balance. A half cup is usually all that is needed.

Oats

For over 100 years, oats have been a mainstay for breakfast and other meals throughout the day. These little grains provide a source of both soluble and insoluble types of fiber that aid the body in the absorption and removal of cholesterol, which is a massive help to heart health.

Studies have shown that people who eat oatmeal have a lower risk of heart disease than those who don't eat it.

Sunflower Seeds

Coronary artery disease is a common type of cardiovascular disease that usually occurs when blockage forms in pathways to the heart. When this blockage reaches the point where it becomes a serious issue the direct result is usually a heart attack. Sunflower seeds and other foods that contain a high level of vitamin E, which has been effective against these blockages, and more effective than vitamin E supplementation. It is recommended to put more focus on antioxidant sources.

Bell Peppers

As a pepper matures through its different stages, the colors become an indication of the flavor that the pepper will provide. The chemical that provides the coloring for the bell peppers are called carotenoids. The carotenoids possess powerful antioxidant properties that help the body to fight cellular damage that lead to a multitude of disorders including heart disease and cancer. They accomplish this by helping to break down the blockages that form in arteries.

These are generally healthy foods that fit a variety of special diets as well.

Top Food Sources of Vitamin B5

Modern medical science has been able to uncover quite a bit of information about the importance of nutrition for the purpose of maintaining health in the last decade. Various studies on which vitamins and minerals support vital life functions in the human body have been published to help document and extend the reach of this life saving research.

One of the most important systems in the body is the cardiovascular system. One of the best vitamins that promotes cardiovascular health is vitamin B5.

How It Works to Help You

Vitamin B5 is a water-soluble vitamin found in a wide range of foods that are common to diets in every culture. It helps to facilitate the chemical reactions that make energy in the human body. It is also an important player in the production of body fat, and helps to create essential hormones. While it's generally understood that few people will suffer from a deficiency of this vitamin, it is possible in cases of low food supply or malnutrition and could lead to some unpleasant effects. The most common of these being muscle cramps, mood swings, and weakness.

Foods That are high in Vitamin B5

This is a list of some foods with the highest vitamin B5 content in order of lowest to highest per 1 cup, with broccoli being the lowest of the group.

Broccoli, cauliflower, sun-dried tomatoes, corn, mushrooms, yogurt, sunflower seeds, salmon, avocados and chicken liver.

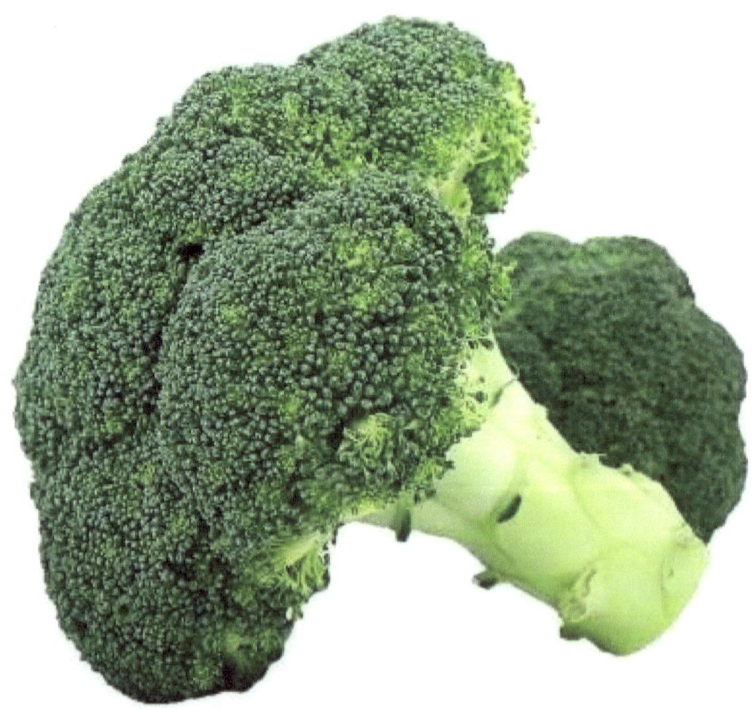

Sunflower seeds, salmon, and avocados contain 20% of the daily value for vitamin B5, but chicken liver has the highest daily value at an unbelievable 83% of your daily value per 1 cup.

Other Positives

Aside from the heart health benefits, Vitamin B5 is also a great help for developing stamina. This can help you to maintain activity for longer periods of time. It is also an effective way to help fight depression. Many of the hormones mentioned earlier in the article that it helps to produce are responsible for chemicals that regulate emotional health and well-being. Keeping a healthy dose of this vitamin in your system may make it easier for you to shake some of those depressive feelings that can sometimes creep into your mind. Grab a few of these to help improve your mood!

Luckily, most B5 sources are also vegetarian and vegan friendly if you are on one of those diets.

Vitamins and Supplements That Help Your Cardiovascular Health

Nutrition that you consume provides you with the raw materials you need to make sure that you can repair your body and grow, so it makes sense that any person would want to be sure that they had the proper nutrition to accomplish that, but today's food landscape is much different than the past. Many people find it very difficult to get what they need without supplementing, and if ignored, this deficiency could cause health issues later. What kind of supplements help with cardiovascular health? Keep reading as this information is geared towards providing you with a short list of some of the most important things you need.

Arginine

This chemical is a naturally occurring amino acid that is good for the heart because it is an important part of the creation of nitric oxide which opens the blood vessels. That means that it has a very positive effect on high blood pressure, and improves blood flow. Studies have proven that taking arginine has the ability to aid vascular functionality, and can limit the effects of symptoms related to cardiac dysfunction.

Fish Oil

The Omega 3 fatty acids contained in fish oil pills is a powerful aid to your cardiovascular health. These amazing pills have been able to cut the triglyceride levels by nearly a third, and have been able to reduce the chances for coronary arterial deaths. Omega 3 fatty acids have also been shown to protect the cardiovascular system against damage by reducing inflammation of the arterial walls. Another amazing side effect is its ability to enhance the erosion of arterial plaque and fats in the bloodstream, making it more difficult for clots and blockages to form.

Plant Sterols

The sterols in plants are structured in a very similar way to the way cholesterol is structured, but if you ingest sterols by eating plants, the sterols block the gut and intestine's ability to absorb as much cholesterol. This has a positive effect on the amount of cholesterol that ends up in the blood stream.

Many organizations centered around heart health have declared that the consumption of plant sterols can help people to live healthier lives and reduce the chances for cardiac incidents.

Lycopene

Although lycopene can be found in a wide range of vegetables and fruits, the tomato has proven itself as the highest and most substantial source of this cholesterol and fat diminishing chemical. It works in the blood to break down clots, arterial plaque and other impurities.

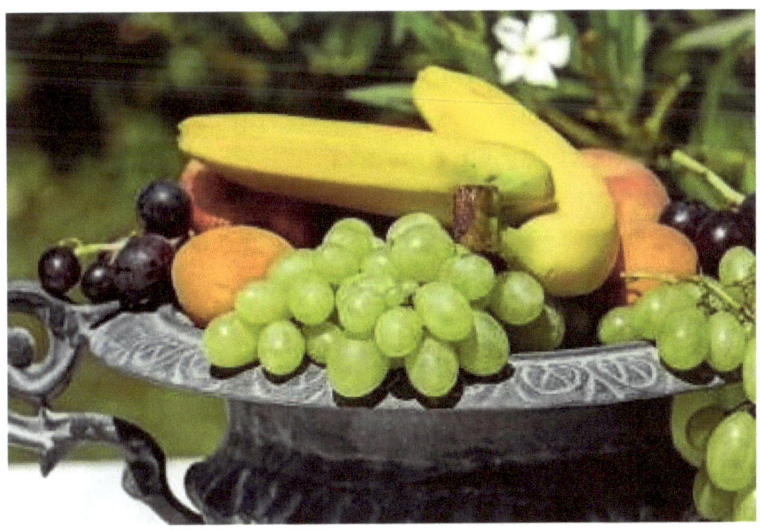

5 Powerful Herbs For Heart Health

Everywhere you look these days there are new fad diets and miracle foods being sold to the public with promises of what they can offer, but what does science say? Fortunately, numerous studies that shed light on how various foods can help people to achieve their health goals, and with that, more knowledge about the role that regular foods play in your health maintenance. Here is a breakdown of a few of the most useful herbs that can help you with your heart health.

Cinnamon

In the last few decades, cinnamon has become a spice that is used in seasonal drinks and treats, but it has so much more to offer. Cinnamon is known for having the ability to lower blood sugar and has powerful antibacterial and antimicrobial properties. The medicinal properties of this spice can make a significant difference in your health and the way you eat food. Studies have shown that adding it to your meal can help to keep your blood sugar from spiking, which is the primary reason that diabetics get damaged organs and arteries.

Garlic

For over 2000 years, this herb has helped people to treat and fight off infections. This powerful antibiotic and antimicrobial herb is packed full of antioxidants and provides a wide range of vitamins to help you heal your body. It has amazing anti-inflammatory properties and has been found to lower cholesterol.

Garlic can be added to a variety of foods for easy consumption.

Ginger

Ginger is a powerful anti-inflammatory that has outstanding antimicrobial properties. Studies have proven that ginger can help prevent blood from clotting which will allow blood to pass through arteries and veins. This can help prevent strokes and other cardiac emergencies. Ginger can be sliced and placed in hot tea to gain many of its amazing benefits.

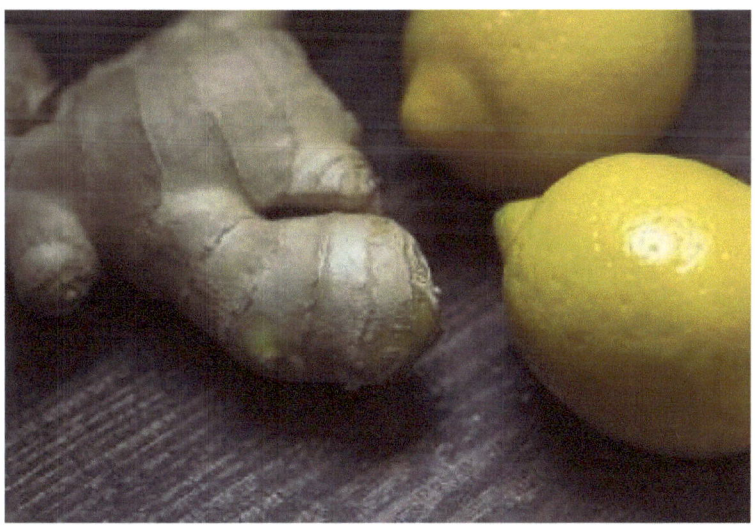

Onion

This herb is known for its strong ability to flavor different types of food. Onion is a powerful antioxidant because of its high sulfur content.

Onions are extremely effective at lowering blood pressure and helping the body to clear harmful fats from the blood stream.

Cilantro

Famous for its heavy use in Indian, Mexican and Chinese food, cilantro is great at preventing cardiac events, and can even help remove heavy metals from the blood stream. It can also speed up recovery from flu symptoms.

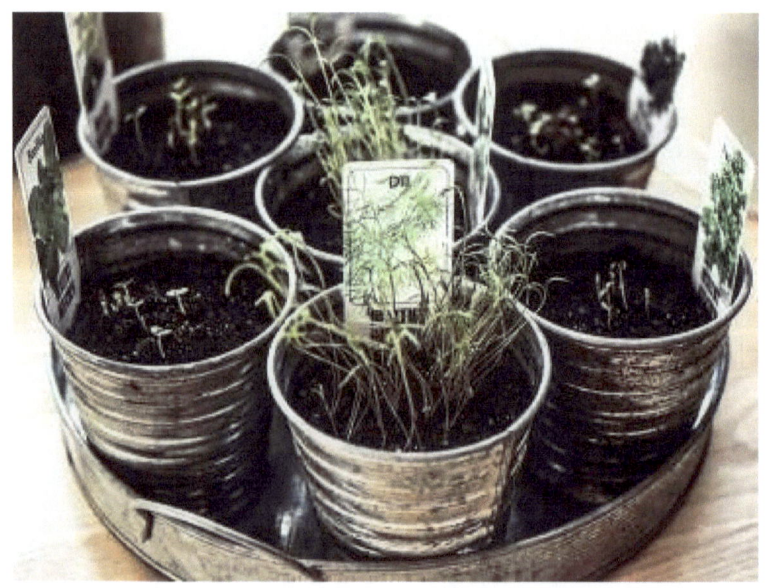

The Impact Exercise Has on Heart Health

In the realm of health, there are an numerous factors that contribute to either good or bad health. Like machines, the human body requires an amount of fuel, and maintenance in order to function at the level that will make it last the longest. For people, maintenance includes exercise. Exercise works to help us achieve a higher level of functionality so we can perform at a higher level when necessary, and function more easily while at rest. The rest of this chapter will be focusing on how exercise affects heart health.

Get Moving

One of the best things for the body is exercise, because as you become more active, your body undergoes changes that help you to adapt to higher levels of activity. The opposite can be said of inactivity, because the converse side of that is the process the body goes through to cut back on supplying resources due to inactivity. This can be very dangerous, because when the heart becomes weaker from not being used, it can put you at risk of heart failure and the cyclical dangers of weight gain. It is never a good idea to go very long without getting your heart rate up.

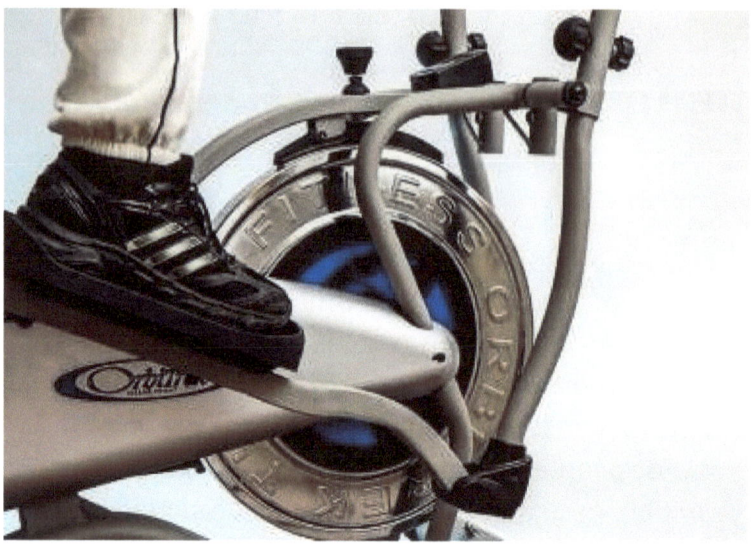

Circulation

When you get good exercise, you are causing more blood to pump through your circulatory system. This in turn works your veins and arteries to help improve their elasticity, as well as helping the body clean itself internally by carrying all kinds of foreign agents and dead cells to waste disposal sites like your lymph nodes. It also improves the amount of fat in your bloodstream (triglycerides), and lowers cholesterol. This leads to healthier extremities, meaning your hands and feel will fall asleep less, and you won't get cold as easily. Cholesterol can be an issue even if you aren't overweight.

High Blood Pressure

If you have been diagnosed with high blood pressure, it's probably a good idea to speak with a doctor before you begin a workout routine.

They will be able to provide you with the kind of exercise that you can do without putting yourself in any sort of danger. When doing any kind of activity, it important to try to maintain normal deep breathing to avoid hyperventilation and still be able to feed muscles the oxygen that they need to function. Know your target heart rate and check it periodically while exercising to make sure you are not overworking your heart.

Exercise is also going to help you lose weight, which as you know can also help with your cardiovascular health.

4 Recommended Workouts For Cardiovascular Health

Making your health a priority takes time, preparation, and perseverance. Some find it hard to stick to a fitness routine, while others seem to thrive when they take ownership of their body, and realize that no one will be there to force them to work out if they aren't able to do it for themselves. One easy way to be sure that you get some exercise in, is to target specific areas one day at a time. This list is designed to share a few simple and easy workout ideas that can help your cardiovascular health.

Fast Paced Walking

Walks can be a very enjoyable way to get your heart rate up for a sustained period of time. Keeping your heart rate up helps to increase stamina, and helps to increase the elasticity of your arteries. A good way to get started is to start off at a slow pace and work your way into a fast-paced walk. Or keep the same pace, but increase the distance. Or add some intensity to your walk by choosing a different route that has some hills on it. The point? Keep it fresh and challenging. Eventually, you will want to up the stakes and begin to do a more robust form of exercise.

Running

It should be obvious that running requires a lot more energy to carry your weight and uphold your stamina. After you have already gotten used to the fast-paced walk, go ahead and try to run. If you can keep up a running pace for awhile, time yourself and see how long you can run before you have to stop. That will give you a new milestone for you to conquer.

Swimming

This aquatic exercise is extremely low-impact, and can burn a lot of calories. A good swimming program can work important muscles to help stay you trim and fit. You can use different exercises on different days to help you work different sets of muscle groups, all within a low-impact, joint-friendly environment thus providing you with a workout experience not available on land.

Try swimming with your fist closed. This will make it harder and you will work harder to get anywhere. You can also try only swimming with only your arms.

Weight Lifting

This workout is not only a fantastic way to get in great shape, but also a way to improve your heart health. When you lift weights your heart rate increases and delivers the oxygenated, life giving blood to more areas of the bod. It's important to remember that you don't overdo it so you can have the opportunity to work out more regularly.

Final Thoughts

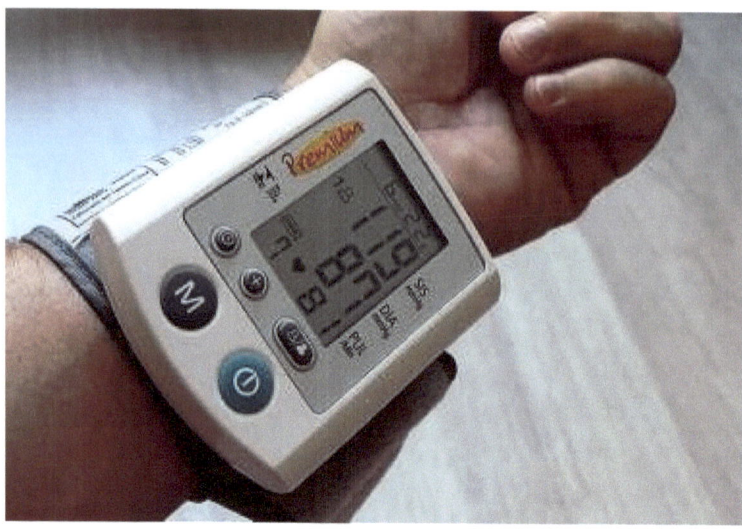

Heart disease is not an illness to lose hope over because there are many prevention and treatment methods available. Simple steps that you can take to prevent heart disease include having a healthy daily diet which contains fiber and complex carbohydrates, exercising and being more active. Moreover, a reduction in the consumption of saturated fat and trans fat will also greatly reduce the chances of having cholesterol build up in the arteries, resulting not only in poor transportation of oxygen in the blood, but eventually what could become blockage.

Heart disease awareness is important and familiarizing yourself with heart disease and the various symptoms will be good in helping you identify the problem before it worsens. Doctors will be able to consult on the condition of your heart and advise accordingly.

Moreover, when you understand the heart disease problem better, you will realize the importance of a healthy diet and lifestyle on your heart's health and hopefully make significant changes to your current one.

Other Relevant Books by This Author

If you would like to read more relevant books about this topic, here is a list of the CreateSpace links, titles and descriptions from this author:

https://www.createspace.com/6435460

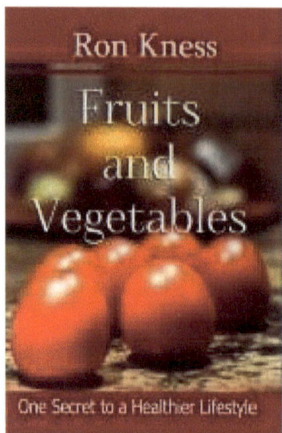

Fruits and Vegetables: One Secret to a Healthier Lifestyle

The way the human body processes food has not changed for thousands of years, however, our predominant food supply has. With the advent of modern agricultural and food processing methods, we have seen a lock-and-step increase in heart disease, cancer and other dangerous and deadly conditions.

That is because modern-day food is unfortunately highly processed. Salt and refined sugar, monosodium glutamate (MSG) and trans fats, preservatives, steroids and man-made chemicals are intentionally injected into most of the food you eat.

This is not done to make you healthier. It is simply done to make the food longer on store shelves, taste better, and to produce as addictive a product as possible (so that you will buy more of it).

Fresh vegetables and fruits (not fried or slathered in unhealthy dressing) have naturally healthy levels of the nutrients, minerals and vitamins your body needs.

They do not contain the processed sugar, insanely high levels of salt, steroids, preservatives and other nutritionally bankrupt chemicals found in processed food.

Unfortunately, the fruits and vegetables that human beings once used to eat in abundance are now lacking in most diets. Your body still craves the same nutrition requirements it did when your ancestors were eating healthy foods.

However, if you continue to reward your hunger with too much unhealthy processed food, and not enough healthy fruits and vegetables, poor health and debilitating medical conditions will be your reward.

The fact that you are a product of nature, and fruits and vegetables are natural food sources, reveals why they are so important as a part of your healthy diet plan.

Another important aspect of swapping out processed foods for vegetables and fruits has to do with how much you weigh. If you find it hard to lose weight and maintain a slim, trim, sexy figure, your diet is probably to blame.

In this book, we explore the fruits and vegetables you should be eating, how much of each you should be eating each day and share some tips on how to increase your fruit and vegetable consumption. Change your diet today and enjoy good health tomorrow and beyond!

https://www.createspace.com/5464020

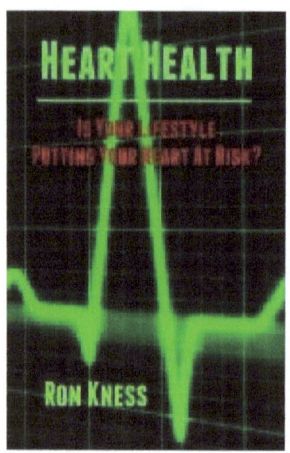

Heart Health: Is Your Lifestyle Putting Your Heart At Risk?

We often take the most important muscle in our body completely for granted. There's only one muscle in our body that never stops to rest. Your heart is an amazing pump that circulates blood throughout your body nonstop.

Your heart actually pumps blood to two separate areas of the body. First, it takes in blood from the body that has used up all of its oxygen. That blood is circulated through the heart to the lungs, where it picks up more oxygen, and then back to the heart. This blood that now has oxygen is then pumped back out into the body to supply your cells with all the oxygen and nutrients they need.

Without a properly functioning heart, your body wouldn't be supplied with everything it needed to work correctly. You wouldn't have the energy you need to keep going. Sadly, many people have heart problems – and most of them can be prevented or even reduced by making changes in your health habits.

It's critical that you take care of the heart that you have. It's one of the most important organs in the body – next to the brain, of course. It has an important job to do and it requires a lot of energy.

There are many ways that you can help your heart to be healthier. The most important things are diet and exercise. But even beyond that you need to make sure that you keep your stress levels low, get plenty of sleep, and keep harmful substances such as tobacco and illicit drugs away from your body.

Your heart is a very complicated organ, but taking care of it can be very simple. You'll need to learn about the best ways to care for your heart. You'll also need to make a commitment to practicing healthy habits.

In my ebook "Heart Health: Is Your Lifestyle Putting Your Heart At Risk?" we discuss the six greatest risks to your heart and the lifestyle changes you can make to mitigate them.

https://www.createspace.com/6988627

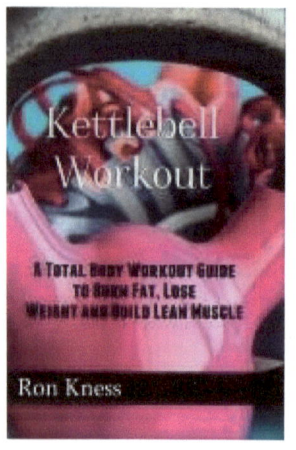

Kettlebell Workout: A Total Body Workout Guide to Burn Fat, Lose Weight and Build Lean Muscle

We want to be functionally stronger - that is building strength that we can use in our everyday lives. We also want to be in charge of our healthy lifestyle. And we want to use kettlebells safely as a workout program!

We can achieve ALL of these goals with the newest release from Ron Kness called "Kettlebell Workout - A Total Body Workout Guide To Burn Fat, Lose Weight And Build Lean Muscle".

Based on these exciting teachings, you will learn about all the dramatic benefits of using kettlebells as exercise and proper nutrition as a way of getting healthy.

This book is built around a very clear, concept: burn fat, lose weight and build lean muscle.
It's not just about how to use kettlebells to burn fat, lose weight and build lean muscle. Having a great fitness level is linked to making smart exercise and nutrition decisions. This is because people living the healthy lifestyle have learned the value and benefits derived from being healthy.

In this book, we look at all of the ways you can improve your own fitness level, starting with strength training using kettlebells. This book will also look at the many other steps that can be taken to support this goal, from learning how to properly lift and swing kettlebells to torching calories from a kettlebell workout.

The choices you make about healthy food and strength training has an impact on your fitness level.

In "Kettlebell Workout - A Total Body Workout Guide To Burn Fat, Lose Weight And Build Lean Muscle", we'll cover all the bases, giving you everything you need to know to properly use kettlebells as part of an overall fitness program.

About the Author

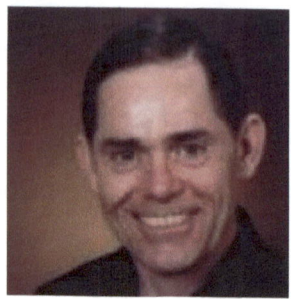

I have published over 125 books on Amazon for Kindle, CreateSpace and other publishing platforms.

While most of my books are on health and fitness in general, as I age (now 65) at the time of this writing) my topics of interest are geared toward aging baby boomers and older.

Besides my own writing, I also ghostwrite ebooks, books, reports, articles, blogs and do Kindle conversions for clients on a variety of topics.

Today my wife and I are retired from our careers and live in Gold Canyon, AZ. I now write as a retirement business where you'll find me happily sitting in my office typing away on my laptop as I work on my next book or ghostwriting project . . . that is if we are not traveling on a cruise ship - our new-found mode of travel.